I'm Hurting,

Not HAUNTED!®

A How-To Guide for Effective Grief Support

L.M.Ivy

**I'm Hurting, Not Haunted!** ©

# Table of Contents

---

# ACKNOWLEDGEMENTS

I have so many people who love me *just because*. They are familiar with my faults (just one or two), my shortcomings (again single digit numbers) and the occasional mood swings (no comment). Some of these incredible people share my blood line like my amazing mother Kathy, my father Jasper, my sister LeKeante, my brothers: Maditchial, Tarunna, Jakamata, McCahte, my cousins (y'all are so awesome), my aunts, my uncles, my handsome grandfather Johney and my dear nieces and nephews.

Others are connected to me by an invisible bond that has survived Orange Grove C.O.G.I.C, M.L.W. Mass Choir (can't wait for the reunion), Felix Mearidy's Bible Study, Kentwood High School (Go Roos!), Southern University, Wellgroup Health Partners, J. Claude Allen C.M.E., New Zion Christian Fellowship, Gift of Hope, LifeGift, New Life and Houston Faith Church.

I am compelled to give a special shout out to a group of women who have played phenomenal roles in my life: Kathy Garret (my mother and my friend), Margaret McCray (the best grandmother in heaven right now), Mercedes L.Williams (for a legacy that will last for generations), Frances Johnson (second mother who loved me like her own), Ann Trappey (one of the best teachers I know), Pamela Bankston (for helping me develop my gift of writing at K.H.S.), Francis Hookfin (my awesome god mother), Brenda Hurst (another second mother who has shaped my life tremendously), Irma Kline (another second mother who can cook like nobody's business), Beatrice Young (for letting me move in and tolerating me and your daughter), Polly Porter ( for putting up with me and your niece), Leola Hookfin (for welcoming me into your home), Valerie Williams (your inspiration is amazing), Mildred Valentine (you know that I love me some you, we still need to start that business), Dr. Kara Davis (First Lady with fire), Helen Ivy (the best mother-in-law ever), Wanda Jackson (beautiful vocals and spirit) and LaShawn A. Williams (you know I have you on speed dial, enough said!). I thank you for pouring into my life and coming to my rescue every time I call!!!

Wallace C. Rials, it started out rough, but I'm grateful that we got to a point where we could appreciate the differences in each other. We miss you dearly, especially A.J. and Adree.

Aunt Willie J. Mearidy, you are my greatest example of what a survivor looks like. I love you dearly!

To my friend who purchased the first copy (you know who you are). I love you to life!

To my mentor, Jackie Lynch, I thank you for taking me under your wings and preparing me for a life time of service to others. The mark of a great leader is one who is transparent enough to lead and humble enough to lift people higher than where he stands. Thank you!

However God's very best expression of His love for me, besides dying on a cross, was putting me in the path of the man He created just for me twelve years ago. This man is an amazing being who models the love of Christ in everything that he does. Andre, I thank you for being my best friend and my lover boy all rolled up into one. The icing on the cake are the gifts that we call Achari, A.J. and Adree. Because of your never ending support, I dedicate this book to all of you.

## For I am persuaded,

- ❖ that neither death,
- ❖ nor life,
- ❖ nor angels,
- ❖ nor principalities,
- ❖ nor powers,
- ❖ nor things present,
- ❖ nor things to come,
- ❖ nor height,
- ❖ nor depth,
- ❖ nor any other creature,
- ❖ shall be able to separate us from the love of God, which is in Christ Jesus our Lord.

**Romans 8:38-39 KJV**

# INTRODUCTION

---

Something brought the two of us together. Come on now let's be real. We are *not* going to sit here and pretend that our lives have been full of rainbows and four leaf clovers. It hasn't been all bad, but it hasn't been all good either. There were some things that happened to you and there were some things that happened to me. My pain might not look like your pain and your pain might not feel like mine, but we both hurt the same. You can be quiet if you want, but I know what I am talking about. If I were in church right now, I would say, "Can I get a witness up in here?" Many of us have been through so much in this life that we have unofficially thrown in the towel. We do just enough to get by because our experiences have left us so depleted. There are depleted parents raising depleted children and depleted spouses who are trying to love on empty tanks. We end up with a bunch of people walking around smiling on the outside, but dying on the inside. If my refrigerator is completely empty and my children are hungry, what is there to give them? When I open the door the only thing on the shelf is water. Because I love my children and want to satisfy their needs, I give them what I have. I may be able to pacify their hunger for a short time, but eventually they will need something more. If I never replenish the food supply, my children will not survive. It doesn't matter that I love them or have a desire to feed them, if I do not meet that specific need, they will die. How can we give our children love when we don't have love for ourselves? How can we promise to spend the rest of our lives with someone when we have never felt worthy of love before? Until we replenish those things that are missing from our lives, we will never experience satisfaction, nor will we ever be able to satisfy anybody else.

Let me tell you about a *friend* of mine. To protect her identity, I will call her "Susie". Susie was a nice girl who worked hard and tried to help people when she could. She followed all of the rules and didn't like to rock the boat. One day (I think that it was a

Wednesday), while she was minding her own business, out of nowhere life hit her so hard that it knocked the wind right out of her. I know you are thinking with your smart self, *"Why does it matter what day it happened?"* Well, there are just some things you do not expect to happen on a day like Wednesday. Mondays and Fridays, you kind of expect for the bottom to drop out. Wednesday is the middle of the week, everybody's defenses are down (Susie's definitely were) and Friday is so close that it makes you get teary eyed just thinking about it. Anyway, back to Susie. She stood there with tears hanging in the corner of her eyes trying to figure out what had just happened to her. She was kind to people, she went to church and she donated money to whoever happened to be standing at the stoplight holding a bucket. What more could she be doing? She knew people who didn't like children or senior citizens and they were doing a lot better than she was. As she sat there in a daze, guess what happened? Life came right back and hit her again. Now let's be honest. Even in a street fight, usually only one punch is thrown and the fight is over. When the guy falls on the ground, there is nothing else to prove. The fight is over (along with the fallen guy's reputation). No one expects for the other guy to jump on the ground and keep throwing punches. Well, this is what life did to my friend Susie. Eventually Susie became so fixated and consumed with life's attacks that she stayed down on the ground and didn't bother getting back up. She stopped loving, she stopped feeling and she stopped being the person that God had created her to be. Susie threw both hands up in the air and screamed, "Life, you win, I.Give.Up!" Then she made the biggest mistake that any of us can ever make in this life; Susie stopped fighting back. She exchanged her chance of victory for a robe of defeat. Susie did what many of us have done; she laid there on the ground and played dead. When life has been so cruel to us, oftentimes it's much easier to just lay there and pretend that we no longer exist. But we know that when we play a role for so long that eventually it becomes part of who you are. Just like Susie, there are teachers and preachers, lawyers and doctors who get up every single morning, putting on nice suits to go and do for others that which they cannot do for themselves. On the outside they are clothed with confidence, but on the inside they are lifeless and barren. Their smiles and their eyes tell two different stories, but only one story is true. At the close of the book, I will share with you how Susie's story ended. You might be surprised. No peeking! I'm sure that we can all agree (you, me and Susie) that life can be so unfair to us sometimes. We constantly pour into the lives of others only to find that we are left empty and unsatisfied. There is one distinct difference between the one who overcomes and the one who is over run. It is a matter of perspective, my dear reader. The overcomer says, "Life has hit me with its best shot, but I am getting right back up. I may be tired, I may be bloody, but I am getting back up." The one who is over run says, "I'm not fighting anymore. What's the use? I'm bleeding, I'm exhausted, I quit." These two people were facing the same adversity (life), but one wins and the other doesn't.

*I'm Hurting, Not Haunted!* is not like the other books you may have browsed through on the shelves. There are thousands of books written by doctors and counselors who filled their pages with outdated *one size fits all* messages and hoped that no one caught on. Much of the information is obsolete and not surprisingly, ineffective. You are not a case study and I will not treat you like you are. You will not find fancy words in here, so put that dictionary right back where you got it from. You will not have to skim over boring philosophical theories or sections that are so deep you need a shovel to dig through them. None of that is in here. I left all of that up to the other guys. I could have easily made this book twice as long, but I wanted this to be a survival guide, not an encyclopedia. The information here is relevant, applicable and life changing. See I have been hurt before and I understand that when a person is desperate to change the course of his life, he needs a fix that is immediate and lasting. This book is a tangible response to those needs. *I'm Hurting, Not Haunted!* is a practical, easy to follow guide that was divinely designed with you in mind. I use plain ole' English (mainly because this is the only language I speak) and a little old fashioned humor to deliver a message that will encourage you who are hurting and inspire you to take your lives back. Not in the great by and by or in that great getting up morning, but right now on (insert today's date). One of the biggest frustrations I witness in my professional career is when well intentioned, but ill-prepared people, try to force feed their "this is the way I've always done it so it must work" beliefs to those who are hurting. Those people withdraw and isolate themselves at a time when they need to be surrounded by family and friends. As the title suggests, there is a stigma that surrounds hurting people and they get treated like they are spooky, instead of wounded. We will tackle those misplaced feelings and get you up to code in no time. You will not only learn about the issues that surround feelings of grief, loss and defeat, but the easy to follow solutions will work for anybody who can read and chew gum at the same time. If you fall outside of that category, let me know and I will send you a book full of shiny pictures. One more thing, if you're the kind of person who likes to go against the grain and do things your way, i.e. start off reading in the middle of the book because starting at the beginning is weird, help yourself. Nobody's judging you here. I designed each chapter to stand independently on its own. Just make sure you go back and read the entire book. It's sort of a big deal for me. I am humbled at the number of pastors and employers in service and support fields who have recommended *I'm Hurting, Not Haunted!* to their congregants and their staff. If that is the avenue by which you have come this way, I am grateful for the opportunity to share with you. Shall we begin?

# NATURAL DEATH & SPIRITUAL DEATH

This chapter will focus on the laws of natural and spiritual death. When we understand these important principles, we are able to live a life that is fulfilling and meaningful. Many people get to the end of their lives and regret "playing it by ear" instead of intentionally living by God's purpose and by His promises. If you are not maximizing the gift of your life, you are doing yourself a disservice and those who are connected to you are getting only broken pieces of you. Things that are broken things are usually unappreciated and undervalued. Only when we know how to live, can we know how to die. We came into this world kicking and screaming because we didn't understand what was happening to us, but we should not leave out doing the same thing. If we do, something is wrong.

I chose this topic first because it will lay the groundwork for understanding how believers of God *should* view death. There are some things in life that are non-negotiable and non-transferable. We had no hand in choosing our skin color, our family or our genetic traits. These things were already in place and we had no choice but to accept them. An inevitable that each one of us will face is natural (physical) death. We cannot bargain with it, we cannot hide from it and we cannot out run it. Its arrival is swift and its presence can linger, but it is coming. We have all witnessed how natural death destroys the looks of beautiful people and transforms the strong and mighty into weak and feeble beings. The wealthiest place in the world (contrary to what the magazines report) is not found in the hills of Hollywood, but in the graveyards that hold great talents like Michelangelo, John F. Kennedy and my all time favorite singer, Whitney Houston. Natural death is selfish, it is prideful and it is boastful. Who else can claim that they have taken hold of kings and queens, the rich and the elite, and billions of others since the beginning of time? Death is indeed all of those things, but even in all of its greatness, it still has limitations. The believer in Christ knows that death can take him, but death cannot keep him. Paul understood this when he wrote, *"O death, where is thy sting? O grave, where is thy victory?"* (I Corinthians 15:55, KJV) It would serve us well to embrace Paul's attitude, *"For whether we live, we live unto the Lord; and whether we die, we die unto the Lord: whether we live therefore, or die, we are the Lord's."* (Romans 14:8 KJV).That tells me that even in the face of death, I am accounted for by the Almighty! Some of my scariest times as a child happened on the playground at Kentwood Elementary School. During the physical education period our class would play soft ball. When it was time to choose teams, I would get nervous because I knew that I wasn't a good player. Both team leaders would scan the class and pick out the people they wanted on their teams. Of course, all of the good players got picked first. I would stand there praying to not be among the last players chosen because it meant that nobody had confidence in my ability to help their team succeed. There were always two people left that no one wanted to have on their team. Usually it was me and another kid who was wheelchair bound. The coach would tell the leaders that they *had* to pick one of us or he would make the decision for them. It was always something along the lines of: "Coach, I don't want her on my team, because she can't run. Give me Sally." Well, all you have to do is look at the front cover to see that my name is not Sally. Yes, they had more faith in Sally and her wheelchair than they had in me! What is the moral of the story? Yes, kids can be mean sometimes, but you are missing the point. The moral of the story is that when death comes knocking at our door, never again will we have to be afraid that no one will pick us or that we will be left standing on the sideline. God has chosen us before the foundations of the world and we are His and He is ours! Let the church say Amen! Look at how Stephen responded in the face of death, *"But he, being full of the Holy Ghost, looked up steadfastly into heaven, and saw the glory of God, and Jesus standing on the right hand of God, And said, Behold, I see the heavens opened, and the Son of man standing on the right hand of God. Then they (his murderers) cried out with a loud voice, and stopped their ears, and ran upon him with one accord, And cast him out of the city, and stoned him: and the witnesses laid down their clothes at a young man's feet, whose name was Saul. And they stoned Stephen, calling upon God, and saying, 'Lord Jesus, receive my spirit'. And he kneeled down, and cried with a loud voice, 'Lord, lay not this sin to their charge'. And when he had said this, he fell asleep."* (Acts 7:55-60, KJV). Stephen didn't beg for his life, nor did he resist the painful position that he had been placed in. Instead he asked that God would forgive those who violently took his life! Stephen's focus was not on where he would spend eternity (he knew where he was going), but his concern was for the very people who took his life! We can learn a lot from Stephen. If anybody had a right to hold a grudge, it would be him. His story completely shatters the theory that forgiveness takes time. If we were to follow Stephen's example, as soon as an offense takes place against us, we would be able to forgive *on the spot*! We don't have to pray about it, set up a meeting with our pastor or ask God to send confirmation after confirmation. Forgiveness sealed Stephen's place in heaven, will it seal ours? Sorry for going off on a tangent, but I believe that revelation is blessing somebody right now. When we understand that death cannot keep us, we can die with dignity. When I come home and step in front of my door, I don't dread going in because I know what's waiting on the other side for me. As soon as I open the door, I know that my husband and my kids will greet me with hugs and kisses. As soon as I see them, I forget about the traffic and all of the challenges that came my way. Why should death be any different for believers? When death comes nigh, we already know what's on the other side of that door; a Heavenly father who is waiting to greet us with hugs and kisses. We will be able to put the cares of this world behind us and know that every pain and every heartache was worth going through in order to get through!

Death is a very small part of our lives, but yet we give it so much credit. It will only last a few seconds or minutes for many of us. (I'm speaking of actual cessation of our heart beat or brain function, not the process of death that can last for months). We spend much more time living, than we will in dying; but death gets the most attention. Something is wrong with that equation. In Philippians 1:21-24 (NIV), Paul wrote to the church, *"For to me, to live is Christ and to die is gain. If I am to go on living in the body, this will mean fruitful labor for me. Yet what shall I choose? I do not know! I am torn between the two: I desire to depart and be with Christ, which is better by far; but it is more necessary for you that I remain in the body.*" Paul recognized that he was facing a win-win situation. Wait... Am I telling you that Paul welcomed death and actually *wanted* to die to be with His Savior? Yes, I am. He was torn between this world and the one that was to follow. I am not insinuating that Paul was suicidal by any means. He saw death for what is was, not as *the end*, but as *the means to an end*. In other words, Paul understood that the only way that he could get to God was by going through death. So death to him was not scary or intimidating, it was just another door that he had to go through in order to reach his goal. Deep stuff, huh? I know many of us who are quick to say, "I want to get to heaven, but just not right now." Is it because we have more faith in this world, than the One who will call us home? Could it be that we are not truly convinced that heaven is as good as the Bible says that it is; otherwise, why would there be such fear and intimidation surrounding death? See Paul understood that the odds were in his favor. If he chose the door on the left and remained in his physical body, he could continue being profitable to the kingdom of God by winning souls. If he chose the door on the right, he would be free from shipwrecks, from being stoned and from unjustified prison time. He would be free to sit at the Master's feet. Though his desire to be in Jesus' presence was overwhelming, Paul understood that it was necessary for him to finish his course here on earth. A very interesting point to consider is that Paul made it clear that it was *his* choice of whether he would remain with the brethren or depart to be with God. Paul asked himself in verse 22, "*Yet what shall I choose*?" Could it be that God allows believers to determine their time here on earth? Before you answer, consider the story of Hezekiah found in 2 Kings 20. Hezekiah was given a death sentence by the prophet Isaiah. Isaiah told him to get his affairs in order because he was *certainly* going to die. Hezekiah cried unto God reminding Him of his devotion and faithfulness toward Him. God was so moved by his prayer that He added fifteen years to Hezekiah's life! Imagine being diagnosed with terminal cancer where literally nothing on earth can be done for you. You turn to God and remind Him of your faithfulness toward Him and how you have brought many into the kingdom by sharing the love of His Son Jesus. God hears your heart and says, "Not only will I heal you of this Stage V cancer, but I will add fifteen years to your life." Is your faith big enough to believe God for a blessing of that magnitude? Notice though, that Hezekiah was able to speak about how he had labored for the kingdom. We don't know if this was God's motivation for extending Hezekiah's life, but God undoubtedly knew that He would be able to count on Hezekiah to continue spreading the good news. Hezekiah had a reputation and a track record that God could count on. Can God count on us? We know that we can count on Him, but can He count on us? Many people seek healing to be able to continue on the same path of setting and carrying out their own agendas. As soon as their strength returns and health is restored, it is business as usual. We must remember that God knows our secret thoughts and the true desires of our hearts. If our prayers are self seeking and shallow, we should not be surprised when there are delays and silence from heaven.

Have you considered how you want the end of your life to look? Will you be tormented by the regret of unfulfilled dreams and unfinished business? Will you be ashamed that you have nothing to show for your life except mistakes, failures and disappointments? A very wise man once said that "to be forewarned is to be forearmed". To put it simple, those who have been properly informed about an event or an occurrence, have the opportunity to thoroughly prepare for its arrival. None of us can afford to be caught off guard any longer; for the choice is ours today. I want to be able to say like Paul in 2 Timothy 4 (KJV), "*I have fought a good fight, I have finished my course, I have kept the faith: Henceforth there is laid up for me a crown of righteousness, which the Lord, the righteous Judge, shall give me at that day: and not to me only, but unto all them also that love His appearing.*" The Bible tells us in Psalms 116:15 (KJV) that, "*Precious in the sight of the LORD is the death of His saints.*"

I don't doubt that there are tears in heaven when a believer transitions from this life to the next, but I believe that the emotional expression differs from the one that we experience here. Instead of sadness and pain, there is great celebration that another child has made it home; never to hurt again and never to die again! When we depart this life, and those we love, we can be assured that our Father is right there with open arms to receive those who are His. This is indeed good news!

# LEARNING FROM LOSS

---

The death of loved ones and failed relationships are among the greatest pains that can be felt in this life; but even in the pain there are lessons that must be understood. The experience of loss becomes costly when people don't allow themselves and others to grieve in a manner that is necessary for them. Some view grieving as an unnecessary weakness and believe that it is "mind over matter"; that as long as they keep thinking that they are okay, they will eventually be okay. That may work for hunger pangs or occasional breakups between you and your fiancé of five years, but it is a no go here. It can be likened to a pregnant woman who refuses to accept that she is pregnant. The signs and symptoms of pregnancy are there, but she chooses to live in a place of denial. She refuses to get prenatal care and she refuses to prepare for the baby's arrival. She ignores the signs that her life is changing and carries on in her ignorance. What she fails to realize is that denial and avoidance does not deter the inevitable from occurring. Eventually the reality of her condition will dominate her fantasy world, forcing her to deal with a situation that would have benefited from early acceptance, planning and preparation. In a similar way when grief from death or other loss is denied, the end results can be dreadful. The brain is a very unique organ. It is capable of hiding unpleasant events and painful experiences in the deep crevices of our minds. However, it is unable to contain those memories indefinitely, and they resurface at inconvenient times. All it takes is just one trigger. That trigger can be a photo, a song or even a fragrance; and the person who put his faith in the "mind over matter" theory, finds himself completely undone. I have seen this happen in restaurants, malls and even grocery stores. People put a great deal of emphasis on funeral arrangements and throwing break up parties, but they neglect to take care of themselves. This is a crucial mistake that must not be overlooked. Allowing yourself time to heal can prevent setbacks that can cost you your time and your mind. Some of you may wonder how I qualify to speak on such a matter, let alone have the nerve to write a book about it. Very good question, I might add. For many years I have stared death in the face. As an End of Life Specialist, I work at Level I, II, and III hospitals supporting families who find themselves in the midst of living nightmares. These families have no warnings and are not given any advance notice. They lose loved ones to gunshot wounds, strokes, drownings, drug overdoses, motor vehicle accidents and other fatal head injuries. I comfort these families during their loss and support them in making end of life decisions that include funeral home arrangements, honoring their loved one's decision to save lives through organ and tissue donation and (probably the most difficult of them all) choosing whether they want to be at the bedside when the ventilator (breathing machine) will be disconnected. I have cried countless tears with these families and am eternally grateful for the opportunity to be invited into such a sacred place in their lives. These experiences teach me things that could never be learned in the finest universities. One of the biggest injustices that I witness is that grieving people don't just suffer from their loss, but they suffer because the people who surround them don't know *how* to help them. Working with these families is a daily reminder that no one is exempt from this place of suffering. And we can all be assured that as we continue on this journey of life, that death is certain for each of us. I heard a preacher once ask, "Death runs in my family, what about yours?" Although it was said lightheartedly, that statement is so true that it is hardly even funny. From the very second we took our first breath, the countdown began. Every now and then as a reminder for me to *work while it is day*, I say to myself, "*Today could be my last day here.*" And the reality is that one of those days, I will be right. So do I let that consume me? Should I pick out my casket, set it up in my house and just wait for death to come? Absolutely not! As ridiculous as that sounds, a lot of people waste their lives doing just that. Instead of a six foot casket set up in their living rooms, they have it set up in their minds. They stop reaching out to people and don't allow people to connect to them. They reason, "*Why build meaningful relationships with people when they are just going to leave me or die anyway?*" There are risks with everything in life and there are no guarantees outside of Christ.

From time to time we will be disappointed, someone will take advantage of us and we will get hurt no matter how careful we are. But the tragedy of you not taking a chance on yourself is worse than all of those things combined. Get rid of the mind casket, it is occupying valuable space and to be completely honest with you, it is just plain weird!

# SHOCK

---

**Shŏk: an unexpected emotional blow that destroys one's sense of security causing vulnerability and defenselessness**

**Meet Theresa...**

I am enjoying a cup of coffee with my husband Bobby on this beautiful spring morning. The birds are flying about and the leaves are swaying as the soft breeze passes through. The two of us are discussing our weekend plans of taking the boat out on the water to enjoy the sun and get in some fishing. I read the list out loud to make sure that I am not forgetting anything. Bobby reminds me to pack the camera and make sure that fresh batteries are put in. Otherwise his brother John will think that he's lying when he brags about the ten pound fish he is sure to catch. We both laugh because Bobby has a bad habit of stretching the truth when it comes to hunting and fishing. If the deer was only 10 feet away, he declares that it was 30 feet. As I update the list, he grabs his keys and kisses me on the cheek before heading out for work. I barely look up as I sit there trying to remember where I left the camera. About an hour later the phone rings while I am packing up the suitcase. The caller on the other end of the phone asks for my name and my relationship to Robert Johnson. I nervously ask what the nature of the call is. A male voice tells me that my Bobby has been in a car accident and that I should get to the hospital immediately. When I try and get more information, he tells me that he is unable to share any further details over the phone. When I get off the phone I notice that I am still clutching the camera in my hand. I grab my keys and head to the hospital. I talk myself out of calling any of our family and friends because I suspect that it is nothing more than a little fender bender and I don't want to get everybody upset over nothing. I arrive at the hospital and am directed to the unit where Bobby is. I sit there in a small room waiting for someone to come in and tell me what is going on with my husband. I imagine that he probably has some scratches and at the worst, a broken limb. And knowing my Bobby, he'll probably choose a hot pink or neon green cast to be able to get a few laughs out of it. The smile is still on my face when the doctor and nurse step into the room. I notice that the nurse places a small box of Kleenex on the table next to me. I figure it is for the next family conference. After introductions, the physician proceeds to share the details of the accident with me. His stern look makes me nervous and uncomfortable. He begins to tell me that Bobby's brain has been severely damaged in the accident and shows me some black and white images on a computer screen. He shows me a normal brain CAT scan then he shows me Bobby's CAT scan. He points out the areas that are swollen and bleeding. Dr. Mitchell tells me that he believes that Bobby's brain has died, but cannot confirm this until a series of tests are performed. He also tells me that Bobby's heart has stopped twice and was restarted with resuscitation efforts. He asked me to consider signing a DNR (Do Not Resituate) order to prevent excessive measures like pumping on his chest and using those paddle things I see on the medical shows, since it still won't change his prognosis. I sit there with my head spinning. How could this happen? Bobby works only 15 minutes from his job. No, this is a mistake. They got the records mixed up. That's it. Bobby's name is so common that they got him mixed up with some other guy. I find myself sending up a prayer for this poor guy's family. His wife has no idea that her husband has been in a horrible accident. My Robert Johnson is at work right now selling computer equipment to clients. I ask the nurse to take me in the room so that I can prove that it is not my Bobby. The nurse leads me into a darkened room and I see my lovely husband of fifteen years lying in the bed. He is bloody, bandaged and hooked up to all kinds of machines. I hear hysterical screaming and realize that the sounds are coming from me. I grab Bobby's hand and tell him to fight, "Come on baby, you have to fight. You can't do this to me, Bobby Johnson. I need you, we need you!" I immediately think about our kids, our precious kids. How do I begin to tell them that just two hours ago we were both having breakfast and now he might not…I push the thought out of mind. I cannot sit still. I find myself pacing from one side of the room to the other. I pick up my phone to try and call people, but my hands are shaking so bad I keep pressing the wrong buttons. The nurse sees my struggle and volunteers to make the calls for me. I sit there in a daze. I am in total disbelief! I reason with myself that this is just a horrible ugly nightmare. I just need to calm down, I'll be awake soon and all of this will be over. We're going to Lake Tahoe this weekend and we are going to have the time of our lives. I cannot wait to tell Bobby how real this dream felt. I can see him now with that big small across his face saying, *"Honey, you know I'm not leaving you; unless of course, Halle Berry ever calls me back."* As soon as I turn back towards the bed, the smile disappears from my face. I can't handle seeing Bobby so helpless. I walk out of the room and go sit in the waiting area. The people in there are laughing and talking. I fight hard against yelling, *"Stop it right now! There is nothing funny at all. My husband is dying and you all are in here laughing like that is okay. Well, it is not!"* But I know deep down that I am envious that their loved ones are doing much better than my Bobby, so I just sit there with my eyes closed for what felt like an eternity. My sister Pat calls my name and I open my eyes and see that quite a few of our family have made it. I try to tell them what has happened, but the words don't make sense. I collapse in their arms. I later walk them to Bobby's room and relive the experience all over again. As I sit there my mind starts playing these awful tricks on me. One second I am hysterical and all over the place. The next I find myself going over the last minute details of our trip in my head. As soon as I realize the nightmare, I become sick to my stomach. I take a mental inventory of all of the things I have ever done in my life to see if I somehow brought this upon myself. Why else would God want to punish me like this? I cannot be a widow at thirty-seven years old. I definitely cannot raise two children by myself. *"God, I'll do anything, just please don't take my husband. I don't care about him throwing his socks and shoes in the middle of the floor and I will never complain about him not cleaning the garage ever again, I just need him back here with me, please God, I'm begging you!"* I sit there and watch the nurse take care of him. I ask her if she's ever seen a person in Bobby's condition survive. She looked up at me after squirting some clear liquid into a bag hanging from his I.V. pole. She told me that in her twenty years as a nurse, she has never seen a person with Bobby's injuries live a meaningful life. Most don't survive and the ones that do require around the clock care and end up being in a vegetative state. She told me that he will probably never be able to speak or laugh or be the person that he once was. She explains that the medication she just started is to keep his blood pressure from dropping too low. Normally the brain controls this, but because of the damage, it has to be done artificially. Her words hit me like a ton of bricks. I feel defeat starting to set in for the first time. My sister Pat grabbed my hand and held it tightly. Over the next few hours, I watch people come in and out of Bobby's room to do consultations and make changes to the machines. Dr. Mitchell came back in to tell me that Bobby was stable enough to have an apnea test performed. He explained that this breathing test would determine if Bobby was alive or not. They are going to draw blood samples, supply him with enough oxygen to sustain him for the test and remove him from the breathing machine for a few minutes. If he took a breath, his brain still had some activity and there is hope. If he didn't take a breath, well, it would not be good. I sit there as they perform the test and for almost ten minutes, Bobby's chest did not move. I am devastated. Dr. Mitchell looks at the shiny watch on his arm and tells me that he is pronouncing Bobby dead at 17: 32. I barely hear him tell me that he is sorry for my loss before I collapse on the floor.

### Meet Amber…

Thank you, God! Thank you, God! I cannot believe that he asked me to marry him. I am so excited that I don't know who to call first. I am a living witness that prayer and faithfulness pays off. I refused to settle for a man who didn't love you, God. If he doesn't love you, how could he ever know how to love me? A pastor's wife…Wow! I never thought that I could be so blessed. Out of all of the women at church, David chose me. What more can I ask for? I have a handsome man who loves God with his whole heart and I get to spend the rest of my life with him. I think about all of the times that I was so lonely that I would cry myself to sleep.

Nobody knew how hard it was for me to watch all of my friends get married and start their families. I was happy for them, God you know that I was, but I wanted the same thing for myself. Then we they got married, all of a sudden their husbands don't want them hanging with me because I was a single woman. Yeah, I was single, but I definitely wasn't no heathen. I tried doing stuff on my own like going to the movies, but the cashiers would give me crazy looks when I would say, "Yes, just *one* ticket, please." I really wanted to tell them, "My husband is overseas fighting for our freedom which is why he can't be here to come to the show with me." I bet that would've wiped that smirk right off their faces, but then I would have to keep the lie going. Instead I grabbed my ticket and hid in the darkest part of the theater. Eventually I started waiting for the movies to come out on DVD, so I didn't have to deal with people who had a problem with *me* taking *myself* out on a date. But since you've blessed me with David, I don't have to worry about any of that ever again. Next year around this time, I will be First Lady Amber Jackson. It has such a nice ring to it. God, thank you for sending my Boaz to me!

**Two years later...**

David is indeed the man of my dreams. This man loves me so much, I can hardly stand it. He sends me flowers for no occasion. It's been two years and he still spoils me with nice things. I am the most blessed woman I know. Ladies, trust me, you don't have to settle for less than what God has promised you. Your king is out there, just be patient and allow God to bring him to you. I have been feeling different the last couple of weeks and I am a few days late. I just took a pregnancy test and it looks like I might be pregnant. Can you believe it? David and I are about to be parents! He is going to be thrilled. We have talked about starting a family and now it looks like it is happening. When God blesses His children, He goes above and beyond what we can ask or think. I have to go to the church to tell David this good news in person. I have to be right there with him. I'm too excited to wait until he comes home. I can see him now walking around with his chest all puffed out. He is going to make an awesome father. Just when I thought it couldn't get any better, look at what God can do! My heart is almost jumping out of my chest as I park the car and walk inside. I see the light shining from under his office door, so I know that he's in there. I take out the plastic bag with the pregnancy test wrapped inside and push the door open. "David, guess what? You are going to be…" "David, what are you doing!?!? Oh my God! Oh my God! David, who is this? Who are you? Get away from my husband! No, David! Why?!?! Oh, my God!!!!!!!

Shock affects a person's memory, perception, rationalization and judgment. People may experience tachycardia (increased heart rate), chest pain and panic attacks. People literally feel like they are going to die under the weight of their pain. Imagine waking up in the morning a wife and going to bed a widow. The foundation that had been solid and steady in Theresa and Amber's life is now filled with potholes and cracks that threaten to pull them completely underneath. They feel themselves sinking and instead of trying to save their lives, they dig their heels in deeper and welcome this opportunity of escape. They conclude that the fight is bigger than the fighter and wait to be carried away on the wings of despair. What makes Theresa and Amber's emotional trauma so devastating is because neither expected that their husbands would be taken away in the manner that they were. Since there were no warning signs, they were unable to prepare for these fatal blows.

**How you can help…**

They both need a strong support system behind them. With the right people in their corners, they can survive this; but it will take time and patience. You cannot expect them out of *your* frustration to just snap out of *it*, because "any other person would be over *it* by now." Granted, your supportive efforts may be exhausting, but you have to remember that you are not there for yourself. You are there (or should be) because they desperately need you. It should not be a conditional offer of support either. For example, you will support Theresa as long as she pulls herself together or you will not support Amber if she decides to take David back. Check your reasons for being there. If you are not sincere and committed to seeing them through their rough times, it will be evident; and most likely best for you to step back until your heart is in it. They both need you to be compassionate. Compassion compels us to overlook our inconveniences for the benefit of others: *"I really don't want to stop by the hospital after work because the traffic is going to be horrible, but I know that Mindy will be thrilled to see me there... I don't want to go by Shana's house today. Since she got divorced, all she does is sit around and act all sad. If she doesn't pull it together, she will find herself not only without a husband, but without a friend!... Sure it may take me all day to prepare a meal for Mike's family, but I know that they will appreciate it since everyone has been so busy planning for the funeral... I don't know why I ever agreed to dog sit for Ralph. Here I am stuck in his house all day while he gets to sit at the hospital with his dying wife. Boy, he really got me good this time..."* Remember that even after your inconveniences, you get to go back home to your happy life, unlike Theresa and Amber. Many of us fall in one of two categories: Either going through a storm or coming out of a storm. We must be mindful of how we treat others, lest we find ourselves alone when the rain starts pouring in our own lives. Lastly, they don't need to be judged. Check your criticism at your door. Their emotions may be all over the place and their behavior may not make sense to you, but they just lost their husbands. You are not there to critique them, you are there to support. Many people don't understand why a grieving mother keeps her son's room the way that he left it or why a widowed husband would rather sleep on his couch instead of in his bed. People need to be free to deal with their loss in a way that is beneficial for them. Your role is to offer consistent and unyielding support. The same way that you would want your own family members treated under these circumstances, should be the motivation for your care toward those who are suffering such a loss.

# GIVE ME PERMISSION TO...

---

This chapter's focus is on letting those who grieve do it in their own way with no rules, restrictions or limitations. These stories will focus on loss from death, but the principles can be applied in other situations. I have had the privilege of working with hundreds of families. They don't look alike, they don't talk alike and they don't grieve alike. I have seen some families throw chairs at walls and tear up waiting rooms because they didn't want to accept that their loved one was gone. I have seen doctors and nurses threatened by a family who refused to believe that nothing more could be done for their loved one. Grief is person specific and should be handled as such.

### "Be Sad"

**Meet Matt...**

I lost my son Ryan six months ago. I remember holding Ryan for the first time. He was so tiny and helpless. I don't know how, but in that moment life changed for me. As I looked into his beautiful brown eyes, I promised him that I would spend the rest of my life being the best husband and father that I could be. There were two births that day, Ryan's and mine. I mark that day as the one when I officially became a man. Words do little to express how amazing it feels to be a father. That little boy had us wrapped around his fingers. From the moment Ryan took his first steps, he would follow me around trying to mimic everything I did. Even as he got older, he still liked to hang out with his old man. Ryan and I were about as close as a father and son could be. Some of my proudest moments as a father were being able to point him out on the field and tell people that he belonged to me. And then all of a sudden, he's gone. This is a nightmare that I do not wish on anybody, not even my enemies. Some days are better than others. Most times I feel like I am barely surviving. I cry for Ryan every day. I miss him so much. I miss not hearing him call my name. I fear that one day I'll even forget what his voice sounded like. I have often heard the death of a loved one be compared to a person who has lost a limb. I hear that even after the amputation, the brain will send signals through the spinal cord as if the arm or leg is still attached. This causes people to feel various sensations (pain, itching) in the area where the extremity used to be called phantom limb, even though it is not there anymore. This explains why I often pick up the phone to call Ryan or drive in the direction of his school and suddenly remember that he is no longer here. We ache every single day for Ryan. He was our miracle baby and he always promised to take care of his mother and me. Imagine having your leg amputated and six months later being criticized for not participating in the 5K run. After all, it's been six months and you should be used to having just one leg now. As absurd as that sounds, it is ridiculous to expect that I should be able to tuck my pain away and pretend that Ryan was never here. Do not make me feel guilty for crying or discourage me from grieving for my son. In my moments of sadness and tears, be supportive by listening and offering a shoulder. Expect that anniversaries, holidays and other occasions will be especially difficult for us. During these times, we may choose to be alone. Respect our decision and allow us to heal in our own way. When we are ready to reach out, we will.

## "Be Angry"

### Meet Michelle...

Last year at fifteen years old my mother had a stroke and died. We had the typical mother daughter relationship. As much as I would love to say that we never had arguments or disagreements, we did. I didn't always obey my mother and there were times when I thought that she was too overprotective. As soon as I became a teenager, I felt like I had all of the answers. Just like any other teenager, I thought that my friends were smarter than my parents. Since my mother's death, I have found myself trying to recall all of the advice that she tried to share with me when I was too stubborn to listen. Unless someone has lost a parent, it is hard to imagine the void that their absence creates. I have found that my mother's death is an inescapable pain that I am unable to fully articulate. I experience many different emotions. One emotion that I am quite familiar with is anger. I remember going into her hospital room to talk to her and hold her hand. I asked everybody to leave the room so that I could be alone with my mother. Out of nowhere, I began to scream at her, "Why would you leave me, Mom? You know that I need you. How am I supposed to grow up without having my Mommy? Who's going to help me pick out my dress for the prom? No, Mom, you can't be dead." My father and one of the social workers had stepped into the room. He tried to get me to calm down, but the social worker told him that I needed to express my feelings. She walked him outside of the room and allowed me to get the closure that I needed. I was grateful that she gave me permission to be angry. I still find myself getting upset when I miss her the most. Last Sunday was Mother's Day and it was difficult for me to just get out of bed. This is the day that I would wake up extra early to make sure that the house was clean and fix my mother's favorite breakfast: scrambled eggs with onions and cheese, bacon and toast. I hated cutting the onions because they always made me cry, but I did it because the smile that would flash across her face was priceless. This year I wanted to still fix her favorite breakfast just to show her that I hadn't forgotten about her special day. But as soon as I picked up the onion I broke down; not from the burning in my eyes this time but from the one in my heart. I threw the onion down and slammed the refrigerator door. My father walked in the kitchen and threw his arms around me. He didn't say a word because he understood. After we held each other for a long time, he whispered in my ear, "MiMi, I know that this is awkward, but can you apologize to that poor onion?" We almost fell down laughing so hard. Since my mother's death, my father and I have a very close relationship. He does not try to be my father and mother and I appreciate that about him. I only had one mother and no one will ever be able to replace her. I will never get over her death and will always grieve for her. My heart aches when I think about my future without her. Her loss will be felt for the rest of my life. She won't be there for my prom, for my high school graduation, through my college years, my wedding or when I have my first child. The pain is so unbearable at times, but I know that she is watching over me, so I want to make her proud. From time to time, I do get upset that all of my friends have their mothers around and I don't. I know that those feelings will never disappear, but hopefully they will lessen as time passes. I am thankful for the people that I have in my life; and I'm grateful that when I am going through these tough moments, they don't judge me.

## "Heal in my own time"

### Meet Chase...

I feel incomplete since Chad died. He absolutely hated me telling people that I was his big brother. I was the oldest by 15 seconds. For some reason, I always saw myself as his protector even though we were the same age. It is strange seeing the ultrasound pictures of both of us. We were like two peas in a pod. We used to tell people that we've been tight from the beginning, and then we'd say *literally* at the same time. People thought that was hilarious. I remember in third grade we both came home crying because everybody kept getting us mixed up at school. We were identical twins in the same classroom (Mom's bright idea), wearing identical clothes (Mom's other bright idea), with identical haircuts (guess who's idea). I told him to stop looking like me and he told me to stop looking like him. I guess that we both had strong arguments. Needless to say from that day forward, I looked like Chase and Chad looked like Chad. It is true that many twins share very unique bonds. We would finish each other's sentences, get random ideas at the same time and even crave the same kinds of food. I miss my brother so much. I keep replaying the accident over and over in my head. The truck struck his side and killed him instantly. I got out of the driver's seat and ran over to him. He was bleeding and wasn't moving. I tried to open the door, but it was stuck. The paramedics arrived and tried to bring him back, but it was too late. I kept telling them to take him to the hospital, but they said that he was gone. They threw a sheet over Chad to cover up his body. All I could think was, *"How is he going to breathe with that sheet over his face like that?"* Mom and Dad arrived on the scene and it was horrible. We were so distraught. That was the worst day of my entire life! Since that day, I have not been the same person. I feel like a shell of my former self. I have tried hanging out with some of our friends, but it just doesn't feel the same without Chad there. I guess I just need more time. I hate when people try and make me feel guilty for not being happy go lucky. There is a reason that I don't want to hang out at the mall. Have you even considered that it might be because Chad and I were going to the mall the day he got killed? Expiration dates are important for food and products like batteries and light bulbs, but not for a heart that has been shattered in a million pieces. My brother and I did everything together. Stop telling me to shake it off and get it together. I beat myself up every day. Chad was supposed to drive to the mall that day, but I grabbed the keys from him and jumped in the driver's seat. I feel so guilty. Why am I alive and why did Chad have to die? I wonder if I had driven a different route, if any of this would have happened. I cannot escape the "what ifs". I'm already hard enough on myself. Trust me, I don't need any help from anybody. Do not make me feel like my life is under a microscope and that everything I say and do will be analyzed. Be careful not to critique and scrutinize my reaction to this storm; because if the same one knocked at your door, you might not handle it as well as you think. Allow people time to heal; and support whatever that looks like. If you don't, you risk people harboring feelings of resentment and anger toward you. Your goal should be to make me better not bitter.

### "Talk about my loved one"

### Meet Harry…

Sandra was the happiest person that I knew. Even as a kid she had a personality the size of Texas. Everyone loved to be around her because she could brighten up a room with just her smile. Now I must admit that there were times when she would put that pretty smile in her back pocket to take care of serious business. I will never forget this as I live. I was riding my home from school when this neighborhood bully named Chris ran up from behind me, pushed me down and grabbed my bike. I had seen what he did to other kids on the block, so I figured getting another bike was much easier than getting my teeth replaced. When I got home, Sandra was the first one who noticed the scratch on my face. I was never a good liar so it didn't take her long to get the story out of me. I begged her not to say anything to our parents and she promised she wouldn't. She told me that she was looking for a friend and asked me to walk with her. We were halfway down the block when we spotted Chris on my bike. My voice was shaking when I told her that it was obvious her friend was not outside and that we needed to turn around and go home. She pointed to Chris and said, "That's the friend I'm looking for." I begged her not to mess with him, but when Sandra made up her mind to do something, she did it. We caught up with Chris and she asked him to give the bike back to me. He said, "Nope, Harry told me that I can have it and I ain't giving it back. It's mine now." Sandra got right in his face and punched him so hard that he fell backwards off the bike. I stood there frozen. I didn't know whether to cry or to run. And then the most surprising thing happened. Chris grabbed his eye and ran off. That obviously wasn't enough for Sandra because she yelled after him, "If you ever come near my brother again, I won't be so nice next time!" On the way back home, I remember thinking that Sandra was the toughest girl that I knew. In my eight year old mind, she was Super Woman. When she was diagnosed with cancer many years later, we didn't give a second thought to her not beating it. She started chemotherapy and radiation treatments and everything looked promising. But the cancer turned out to be more aggressive than the doctors realized and it eventually got the best of her. It is still hard for me to believe even now that cancer won out over my big sister. After a person passes away, many people find it necessary to restrict all conversation regarding them. I think they do this believing that it helps us heal faster, almost like an out of sight, out of mind concept. But the truth is that I want to talk about Sandra and actually want to hear stories about her. Right after the funeral, one of her friends shared a story with me that made me smile. Lisa and Sandra had gone to college together. One night while they were hanging out Lisa spotted a cute guy. She was too nervous to talk to him, so she sent Sandra over to get his number. Well, you can imagine how shocked Lisa was when Sandra came back over and told her that the guy Mike had asked her out instead. Lisa was upset with Sandra for about a week. Sandra went out with him and found out that Mike did not work, had no car and lived at home with his mother. Sandra handed Lisa Mike's number and said, "You wanted his number, you can have him." They both fell on the floor laughing. I thrive on stories like these because it helps to keep Sandra's memory alive. Even if the story makes me cry, it does not mean that I am upset or angry. I am grieving and crying is just a part of that process. Sometimes I even refer to Sandra in the present tense. For example, "She *is* the best cook that I know. She *is* able to take simple ingredients and make a gourmet meal." I am not suffering from memory loss or in denial about Sandra's death. Sometimes the pain of using past tense to refer to my big sister is too great for me at that moment. This is just a coping mechanism for me. Allow me the opportunity to talk about my sister and know that it is okay to share stories about her with me.

### "Let Go"

**Meet Tony…**

Have you ever walked into a room filled with people and only one person stood out to you? That happened to me the first time I laid eyes on Cynthia. I had been shy most of my life and only went out with girls who approached me first. I'm not a bad looking guy, I would just get nervous around really pretty girls. That entire evening, I tried as best as I could to stay close to her. If she went to the Ladies Room, I just so happened to be going to the Men's Room at the same time. As the night wore on, I noticed that this pretty girl would have the same guy walk up to her and he would start chatting with her and her friend. I had never seen him before, but that night I declared him my enemy. How dare he make the girl that I was in *mental* relationship with, smile and laugh so hard? The nerve of him! When I saw him alone, I walked over to him and made small talk. I needed to see how serious they were. I started telling him about my band and I found out that he played the drums. He told me that he always wanted to play the guitar like me. I wondered what he would think if I told him that I would give free guitar lessons in exchange for his girl. We talked some more and I asked if he had come to the party with anybody and he said, "Yes." I thought, *"This is not going well at all."* He said, "Let me introduce you to my girlfriend." Before I could react, we were both standing in front of pretty girl and pretty girl's friend. I thought for sure that my heart was going to jump out of my chest. He tells them, "This is Tony, he plays guitar for a local band." Then he says, "Tony, this is my girlfriend Samantha and this is my big head sister Cynthia." I could not believe it! The big head girl, I mean the pretty girl, was his sister and not his girlfriend. Cindy and I spent the rest of the night talking as if we had known each other forever. I even confessed to her that I had been eyeing her the entire night. She had concluded that I was either a stalker or really thirsty, since I kept refilling my drink from the bar that so happened to be where she and Samantha were standing. We both laughed. Since that night ten years ago, we had been inseparable until a year and a half ago when she passed away. I am a fire fighter and have been trained to handle devastating situations. But when I lost Cindy, all of that training went right out the door for me. One of the most difficult parts of losing Cindy was letting go. I remember how I would sit at her bedside day in and day out. I refused to go home because I feared that she would wake up and not recognize any of the hospital staff. No matter how much the nurse assured me that they had my contact numbers on file, I refused to leave the hospital. I was clinging to my hope that the nightmare would be turned around; and when it did I wanted to be right there so Cindy would know that I never left her side. You can't imagine how hard it was when there was no more hope to cling to. Once the doctor pronounced her dead, I struggled with not being able to take her back home with me. I felt like I was betraying Cindy by leaving her behind. I remember the nurse sharing with me that when the time came to let go, I would feel it in my heart and my job at that moment was to allow Cindy to be released. The nurse made it clear to me that I was not walking away from her, but by releasing her I would be able to honor and cherish her memories and our life together. I found this to be a great source of relief for me. I realized that I just didn't know *how* to let go and was given permission to do so in a way that was befitting to my beautiful wife. That moment was liberating for me and became the first step I took in my healing journey. I miss my pretty girl, but find comfort in knowing that she is not in any pain and that I will see her again one day.

# I'M HURTING, NOT HAUNTED!

---

When I started writing this book, I knew that it was important for me to design a cover that was an accurate representation of the stigma attached to people suffering from loss. As the book cover suggests, hurting people are treated like they are frightening instead of victims of circumstance. I have seen sex offenders get better treatment than someone who has lost a loved one. The tragedy is that this shunning is done at the hands of those who call themselves a friend. Many people are just uncomfortable with death or dissolved relationships, so instead of embracing people, they push them away; not considering that their actions are hurtful and cruel. When a couple breaks up after a long relationship, people feel like they have to pick sides. For some reason, they think that if they stay close to both parties, they are somehow being disloyal. So it becomes a personality contest. They embrace the one they like the most, even if that person caused the break up, and pull away from the one who may have been abused or cheated on. That makes about as much sense as plus sized skinny jeans. There goes that "mind over matter" theory popping up again. "If I think that I'm skinny, then I will be skinny." I have tried that one for years. I'm a lot of things and skinny is not one of them. Stay focused, people, we have a lot more material to get through! Anyway, people don't mind coming around as long as there is a crowd. This explains why there is such a presence after the news of a death gets out and during funerals. But as soon as the last plate is served at the repast or the break up party, people scatter like pimps during a raid. I have even heard of people taking a different route home or going out of their way to not come in contact with grieving people. You would rather drive across town to pick up a gallon of milk than go to the corner store that is practically in your backyard. Pete's great-great aunt died last week and you are afraid that he might be working the front counter today. There are a few possible options here: 1) Maybe Pete is off today. 2) He could be out to lunch. 3) He could be in the back stocking tissue and toilet paper on the shelves. 4) Pete could not have even liked his aunt Emma Jean, so no harm, no foul. But no, you are convinced that poor Pete is standing outside in the parking lot flagging down people, so he can cry on their shoulders. It is also interesting how people feel like they have to be deep and profound when they speak to those who are hurting. All of a sudden "Good Evening" becomes too shallow, so they replace it with, "I pray that thou art faring well on the eve of tomorrow" or instead of saying "I'm sorry about your divorce, I'm praying for you" they feel compelled to say something like, "I will beseech the One who sitteth on the throne to givest thou an abundance of comfort and peace during thy troubled time". Unless you are trying out for a part in a Shakespearean play, it is probably not a good idea to use words (in any setting) that you don't fully understand. Something else that happens way too often is when people charge those who are grieving with the task of calling *if* they need anything. Many people do it because it makes them look notable; then they secretly hope that their services are not requested. Remember that those who are hurting are overwhelmed and already have a lot on their plate. It would be more beneficial if you volunteer to meet a specific need like mowing the lawn, dropping a dish off or putting some money in a card. This is how it usually happens: (you must use a Southern dialect for this to work), "Janie, now you call me if you need anythang, and Janie (they pause about six seconds for emphasis), I do mean anythang. Me and Skeeter been friends since Heck was a puppy. Im'ma shole' miss that old rascal." If anybody knows who Heck is and how long he has been a puppy, please write me at hurtingnothaunted@gmail.com.

On a serious note, I want you to hear Barbara's story. I'm sure that she can teach all of us a thing or two about overcoming these insecurities.

**Meet Barbara...**

When my daughter Vicky passed away, we were flooded with people checking on us constantly, dropping off food and donating money to help with her funeral expenses. We were overwhelmed that so many kind people would bless our family the way that they did. I was in such a fog that I was barely able to put one foot in front of the other to even walk. It was such a relief to not have to worry about cooking or cleaning. We were able to plan the funeral and put our baby to rest. After the funeral, all of that changed. People stopped checking on us and the phone calls dried up. It's as if the unspoken message was *"We got you through the funeral, now you're on your own."* The eerie silence in our house is a painful reminder that Vicky is gone. I miss her laugh. It was such an infectious laugh. Even if the joke wasn't funny, people would laugh just because she was laughing so hard. Since Frank has gone back to work, I am alone in this big house by myself. It would be nice to have someone call and tell me that our family is still in their prayers. People avoid me like I have leprosy. I will go out shopping and I notice that people act weird when they see me. I actually saw a person who I thought was a good friend duck behind the aisle so I wouldn't see him. You would have thought that I was someone from the IRS. Well, it was hard for anybody *not* to see him standing there with canned corn rolling off the shelves right next to him. I must admit that I got a chuckle out of that, but it still hurt. I guess people think that if they talk to me in public that I will break down crying and make an embarrassing scene like John did in the canned vegetable aisle. I thought that I was the only one until Frank came home and told me that a few of the guys at work started taking earlier lunches to avoid having to eat with him. These are the same guys who come over to our house to watch the game when their team is playing. It broke my heart when he said, "Boy, you find out who your real friends are when you go through something." It is so upsetting to see people whispering things to each other when they see me. I'm sure that they're saying, *"That's the girl's mother right there, you know the one who was killed in that big accident on Hwy 10."* I wish that people were not so rude to us. Stop treating us like we have Mad Cow's Disease. Stop pretending that you don't see me and when you do, that you're in such a big hurry. I am still the same Barbara, not some weird or freaky person. I lost my baby in a horrible accident and as much as I wish that I could change that, I can't. I could really use your support. I am not expecting you to be Dr.

Phil, I just need to know that you are there for my family. Please stop isolating us at a time when we need to be surrounded by family and friends. Your generosity and thoughtfulness contribute to our healing and inspire us to move forward.

# SILENCE SPEAKS VOLUMES

Not only does loss make some people act weird, it apparently makes them put both feet in their mouths. In the previous chapter, I talked about how people believe that there is an unspoken expectation for them to use fancy words in difficult situations, believing that true comfort is given by using eloquent phrases and being deep like Gandhi. They are convinced that if they say the *right things* that people will somehow be transformed into a less hurting state. This is simply not true. Healing is not going to be immediate when a person has lost a loved one or a close relationship. It takes time and prayer. Some people are uncomfortable with silence, so they try to overcome it by filling the air with random conversation. Instead of them just sitting there, they start talking about whatever comes to their minds. They ask inappropriate questions like, "You must have done something to make her cheat on you" or "Aren't you excited everyone's coming home for your sister's funeral?" These are horrible things to say. Do *not* let your uncomfortable feelings cause you to speak without thinking. You can cause more damage to someone who is already devastated. Words are like feathers on a windy day; once they are gone they can't be taken back. As the adage states, "Silence is golden". Do not underestimate the power of your presence. A hug will go a lot further than a thousand words spoken unwisely. I have spent many silent hours in bereavement rooms at hospitals just sitting there holding a person's hands and rubbing their shoulders. If they chose to speak, I acknowledged what they said. Some people are not comfortable with hugs and kisses, so a handshake may be more appropriate. Pay attention to how they respond to other people. Otherwise, you could find yourself on the wrong side of the law.

I have taken the time to compile a list of the most inappropriate and offensive things that have been said to people in these situations. Sadly, many of us have been guilty at one time or another. If you have been the offender, please raise your right hand

and repeat after me. "I, (insert name), promise to never speak again without thinking, no matter how uncomfortable I am. I choose from this day forward to say what I mean and mean what I say." You can put your hand down now. Thank you.

**Cliché #1 "I bet you're glad to be divorced? You are a free woman!"**

*What the hurting person thinks*: "When I got married my intention was to only do it one time. I'm hurt and I'm devastated. That is a long way from being glad."

*How the hurting person usually answers*: "I'm just taking it one day at a time".

**Cliché #2 "You should be happy, your loved one is in a better place."**

*What the hurting person thinks*: "Happy? I should be happy that my husband will never see our kids grow up and finish school. The better place as far as I'm concerned was right now with his family."

*How the hurting person usually answers*: "Yes, I guess you're right."

**Cliché #3 "I know how you feel losing your wife."**

*What the hurting person thinks*: "How can you possibly know how I feel? I just saw Tammy and she looked fine to me, you insensitive jerk!"

*How the hurting person usually answers*: "Yeah, it's tough".

**Cliché #4 "There are other fish in the sea. Next time just catch a better one."**

*What the hurting person thinks*: "I just found out that the woman I love does not love me anymore. She left me alone to raise our kids by myself, and all you have to say is 'pick a better fish', how about I punch you in your face, so you can pick your teeth off of the floor?"

*How the hurting person usually answers*: "You're right, I'm sure there are."

## Cliché #5 "You're both young, you can always have more children."

*What the hurting person thinks*: "I can have ten more children and all of them together would not replace my child. Imagine your little Annie being snatched away from you, how many kids would it take to replace her?"

*How the hurting person usually answers*: "Yeah, we'll see."

## Cliché #6 "Some things just aren't meant to be."

*What the hurting person thinks*: "My fiancé just died and you have the gall to say this to my face! We were supposed to be married in four months and you tell me that some things just aren't meant to be? I'm very upset right now and if you knew what was good for you, you'd get out of my face! I can show you a thing or two about what's not meant to be."

*How the hurting person usually answers*: "Maybe not."

## Cliché #7 "Well, at least you lost *it* early. It's not like *it* was a real baby."

*What the hurting person thinks*: "From the moment I found out I was pregnant, my baby was real. She was so real that she had a heart beat and fingers and toes. I didn't just imagine carrying a baby for five months. How insensitive!"

*How the hurting person usually answers*: (Just stares in disbelief)

## Cliché #8 Look on the bright side, you hadn't talked to him in years.

*What the hurting person thinks*: "That may be true, but it doesn't change the fact that he was my father, you Moron."

*How the hurting person usually answers*: "Yeah, we did lose touch for a couple of years."

**Cliché #9 "At least she didn't suffer."**

*What the hurting person thinks*: "How do you know that she didn't suffer? Have you ever been thrown out of a car going 60 M.P.H.? Unless you have been through that and lived to talk about it, I suggest you take that nonsense somewhere else."

*How the hurting person usually answers*: "I hope not."

**Cliché #10 "You need to stop acting like this; you have other people depending on you."**

*What the hurting person thinks*: "I apologize for not being the life of the party lately. Not sure if you remember, but my wife left me and took our kids with her. I have not seen my kids in six months. Do you know what it feels like to not know where your kids are?"

*How the hurting person usually answers*: "Acting like what? Like I miss my family!

# CHILDREN & DEATH

---

Death is a hard concept to grasp even for mature adults. Imagine having many of your life experiences taken away, along with intellect and reasoning; then forced to deal with something as overwhelming and dreadful as death. Well, that's how death is for a child. Many times when death occurs, adults may overlook the children affected by the loss believing that they shouldn't be exposed to it. Oftentimes assumptions are made that kids will somehow figure it own on their own, as some adults may have had to learn in their own childhoods. But the truth is that children need to experience the effects of death and have a healthy understanding of it. I have seen times when adults chose not to share a loved one's death with children because they believed that they would not be able to handle it. I believe that this is an injustice for children because when they question where that person is, they are robbed of the truth and the experience. The truth is that children are very resilient and need to know that death is a natural part of life. I want to share Robby's story with you so that you can understand the importance of this concept.

**Meet Robby…**

My name is Robby and I am almost seven years old. Every Sunday me and my sister Ariel and my Mommy and Daddy would go to NaNa and Big Daddy's house for dinner. I got to eat all of the ice cream that I wanted as long as I ate all of my dinner. One day NaNa got sick and had to go to the hospital. Something happened to her heart and the doctor couldn't fix it, so NaNa went on a faraway trip (maybe like Paris) and she is not coming back. When Daddy told me this, he was crying. I told him, "Daddy, don't cry, when I get out of school, we can all go and visit NaNa." But he told me that we couldn't go because she was so far away. He said that she had called last night when I was asleep and wanted them to tell me to be a good boy and to be nice to Ariel. I am very sad because I miss NaNa. I wish that she would have taken me with her. Since she left, Big Daddy is coming to stay with us for a while. I guess that he is sad, too. When I grow up, I will get on a jet or an airplane and fly to see NaNa. She will be so happy and me, too.

Sadly, Robby's story is not uncommon. Instead of him being given the opportunity to have a healthy understanding of death, he is fed untruths. Robby is likely to develop feelings of resentment toward his grandmother because she left on her trip without even telling him goodbye. He might even question if she loves him, why else would she just leave him like that? Robby is likely to develop feelings of insecurity and inferiority. Can you imagine the betrayal that he will feel towards his parents when he finds out the truth? I have seen my share of children trying to cope with the death of a loved one and it is devastating. But at least these children are afforded the opportunity of closure.

Adults need to be extremely careful about how death is explained to children. I remember a particular case where the parents thought it best to tell their young child that his grandfather was sleeping (dead), but that he would never see him again. Well, I was not shocked to hear later that this child was terrified of falling asleep, as he believed that he too would go to sleep (die) and never be seen again. We must remember that children are very literal and will take what we say at face value. I have a perfect example of this. When my maternal grandmother passed away, my husband and I sat down with our two young children. We shared with them that their Granny had died and that she was in heaven with God. Well, on the day of the funeral, my seven year old daughter asked me, "Mommy, are we going to heaven today?" I gave her a puzzled look and asked why she thought that we would be *going to heaven*. She said, "Because you and Daddy told me that Granny was already in heaven." Needless to say, additional conversations took place and we learned that with children, you mean what you say and say what you mean. I must also mention that extreme caution should be taken when considering whether children are capable of handling certain things. Some of the families want their children to go into the hospital room to see their loved ones for the last time. You must remember that a great deal of deaths are from traumatic events, so there could be a lot of swelling, bleeding and deformities that even adults have a hard time viewing. A few of the hospitals have programs in place where trained social workers sit down with the children to assess their maturity before exposing them to these situations. They use dolls to help explain the tubes and equipment that their loved one is attached to. This helps to prepare the children for what they will see when they are allowed to go into the room. Unfortunately, most hospitals do not have this program in place and I have to sit down with the families and help make that determination. Some adults even try forcing their children to go into the hospital rooms believing that it will bring them closure, even when the children are adamantly opposed to it. I stress to the parents that once the children see their loved ones in that condition, they will keep those images in their heads forever. If they are not mature enough to handle it, they could have major problems in the future. There are adults even today who have images in their heads from childhood that still cause deal them a great deal of anxiety. Remember that no one knows your child like you do. Sit down with him and assess his understanding of what has happened. After a close death or divorce, you may notice behavioral changes in your child. Acting out is one of the most common reactions that a child exhibits in these situations. They can become rebellious, defiant and disobedient. As the adult, it is imperative that you take a step back and realize that beneath all of the negative behavior is a child who is hurting and trying to cope with the loss of a special person. A child who was previously happy and fun-loving may become withdrawn and introverted after the loss of a loved one. If this continues, the child may be struggling with depression. Seek professional help immediately. In some cases, medication and therapy may be needed in order to restore proper balance. Counseling is a very effective tool that can measure the impact that the loss has had upon a child's mental and emotional state. I have noticed in my profession that children are sometimes more comfortable sharing their feelings with strangers than with those closest to them. And that is okay. The goal is to get them to a better place. Their survival is dependent on the love and support given to them by the adults in their lives. Exercise patience and love, and understand that with the right support, this too shall pass.

# DIVORCE

---

## Meet Melissa...

I had the perfect life. I was married to a wonderful man with three beautiful children; twelve year old Tyler, eight year old Kaitlin and five year old Danny. We took yearly vacations when our budget allowed for it. We went to church on Sundays and even Bible Study on Wednesdays. I was a stay at home mother who took pride in keeping the house together. My husband Marc owns his own car repair shop. The business has done well the last two years and we were thinking about opening another shop across town. The kids got along like typical kids; one minute they played well together, the next they were screaming and yelling at each other. Our picture perfect family was shattered three months ago when our baby Danny drowned in our pool. My heart bleeds when I think about how scared and lonely he must have felt struggling to stay alive. Somehow he slipped outside unnoticed and jumped into the deep end of the pool. Usually the gate remained locked, but that day it wasn't and we all are suffering from that consequence. Nothing in this world prepares you for finding your baby lying face down and motionless in water. It is a sight that consumes my mind every minute of my life. CPR was useless, he had been in the water for too long. Marc rushed home and we all hugged each other for what felt like hours. The next few days felt like an out of body experience for me. My movements were slow, my thoughts were sluggish and I felt completely out of sync with the rest of the world. Not much has changed in three months. I see that Tyler and Kaitlin are suffering and I want to reach out to them, but I don't know how. It takes everything in me just to get out of bed in the mornings. Some days I don't make it out. I feel like I am buried alive dying a slow painful death. Marc has gone back to work and we barely see each other. By the time he makes it home, I am asleep or crying in our bed. When he has tried to console me, I have pushed him away. He cried when Danny first died, but lately I have not seen him show any emotion. I resent him for not hurting the way that I'm hurting. We barely talk to each other and when we do the words are ugly and belittling. I found out a couple of weeks ago that Marc was the one who left the gate unlocked to the pool. I am so angry with him. If he had locked the gate, Danny would be here right now. I can't believe that he would be so irresponsible and not protect our baby. I cannot believe that I married someone so careless! And to top that off, he wants to be intimate with me. How can he think about something like that when our son is dead? It has only been three months. He is selfish and only thinking about himself. I guess that I should not be surprised since he seems to be doing so well these days anyway. I begged him to take some time off, but he insisted on going right back to work. Apparently his job is more important than his family. I refuse to stay married to a man who selfish, inconsiderate and irresponsible.

**Meet Marcus...**

Even as a little boy I knew that I wanted to have children. I was an only child growing up and I hated not having brothers and sisters to play with. My parents told me that I was such a wild child that I messed up the chances for anybody else to come along. Don't get me wrong, being an only child had its advantages. I never had to wrestle for the remote control, I always got the prizes out of the cereal boxes and I never had to share my room with anybody. Still there were times when it would have been nice to have somebody to boss around. When Melissa and I started getting serious, I asked her if she wanted to have children. She said, yes, but only one. I figured I would be able to use my charm to get her to have at least one more if we ever decided to get married. About two years later, we did get married. In that second year, we welcomed Tyler into the world. Boy, did he have energy. Many times we found him standing up asleep in his crib with his head leaning against the rail because he fought his naps so hard. He kept me and Melissa on our toes. After some hardcore begging, and a nice piece of jewelry, I convinced Melissa to have one more child. I promised her that it would be a girl. God must have seen that I was in way over my head and granted this request for me. Four years later our little Princess came along. She had the brightest eyes that I had ever seen for a newborn. She looked around the room with an awareness that seemed strange for a person who had just come out into the world. I have been smitten since that moment. Kaitlin loves playing dress up and is convinced that being a professional princess is as reasonable as one growing up to become a doctor or lawyer. The kids were healthy, the business was just starting up and Melissa and I couldn't get enough of each other. Life was great! I scheduled the appointment to get my vasectomy content with our family of four. Two weeks after the procedure, Melissa found out that she was pregnant. We were in complete shock. Once the kids found out, we couldn't help but get excited because they were thrilled. It's amazing how we think that our lives are great just the way they are until something comes along that makes it even better. That something was our Danny. Danny Boy came on the scene and completed the circle for us. It is amazing how a tiny and toothless baby can have you in the palm of his little hands. Danny had always been a curious child which is why we installed the gate leading out to the pool. He was our little explorer who always came up with unbelievable ideas. He wanted the sun and moon to switch places so that he could sleep during the day and go to school at night. June 25th changed everything for us. It started out a typical day for me. I left early for work to get a head start on business for the day. Everyone was still in bed when I left. Hours later as I was rotating tires, my secretary Theresa screamed for me to come to the phone. I could tell by her tone that something was wrong. All I remember is Melissa screaming that Danny wasn't breathing. I must have made it home in ten minutes instead of the usual twenty that it took. When I got there, the paramedics were doing CPR. It killed me to see my baby's blue lifeless body being banged on so hard. I told them to stop, we all knew that he was gone. I can't remember how we got through the funeral, but somehow we did. I can't stand seeing Melissa sobbing all hours of the day and night. When I'm by myself I cry, but I try to be strong for Tyler and Kaitlin. Melissa has shut us all out and I need to keep them going as best as I could. I felt trapped inside of that house, so I went back to work. I intentionally work sixteen hour days to not have to see my family fall apart. Many days I come home and see Melissa in the same spot where I left her hours before. The kids spend most of their time in their rooms. Tyler shared a secret with me a few weeks ago. He admitted that he was the one who left the gate unlocked. He feels horrible. I told him that we all make mistakes, but he still feels so guilty. About two weeks ago, Melissa confronted us demanding to know *who* had left the gate open. She was screaming at the top of her lungs. Tyler looked so scared and my heart melted for him. Like any good father, I wanted to protect him. So I told Melissa that I had left the gate unlocked and that is was my fault. I didn't think that our marriage could sink any lower, but it did. I see the hatred in her eyes when she looks at me. I would rather deal with her wrath than have Tyler feel any worse than he already does. I just wish that I could hold my wife. I miss her so much. I want us both to fight, but lately neither of us have the strength to even get in the ring.

I wanted to add this chapter in the book because many people do not realize the impact that death has on a relationship, especially when it is the death of a child. This is one of the hardest challenges that a couple can face. What oftentimes happens is that both parents are so consumed in their own grief that they are unable to reach out to their spouse to give support or receive support. Both parents subconsciously start focusing on their own state and neglect the need and care of the other. As time passes, the separation widens and the relationship begins to suffer. Communication becomes ineffective and the marriage starts to deteriorate. Usually when this happens, people start lashing out at each other because they would rather argue and fight than to have all of those intense feelings bottled up inside. Melissa accuses Marcus of not loving their child as much as she did because he seems to be getting along just fine without him. She is appalled that he could even think about intimacy at a time like this. Marcus accuses Melissa of neglecting their other two children who are alive and need their mother. He also reminds her that he needs his wife back. Underneath all of the bitter words are two people who don't know how to effectively support the other, so they find independent ways to cope. This can be in the form of an adulterous relationship, turning to drugs and alcohol or other distractions. Instead of coming together sorting through their feelings, both parents justify their positions and blame the other for the downfall of the relationship. Something else that often happens after the death of a child is one parent becomes over protective of the remaining children. This causes additional stress on the family resulting in frustration for everyone. If counseling is not sought after, separation or divorce is imminent. Do not try and handle this alone. There are many wonderful people out there who can provide you with tools and techniques to help you cope with your loss and help strengthen and rebuild your marriage. No parent ever gets over losing a child. With the right support, you can learn to adjust to their absence and honor them by moving on.

# COPING WITH SUICIDE

---

One of the hardest deaths to cope with is suicide. I have seen many families devastated by this type of loss. There is usually a lot of guilt associated with suicide. People wonder if the outcome would have been different had they come straight home instead of stopping at the store or if they had not missed the phone call or if they had paid attention to the warning signs. The guilt is consuming and stands in the way of their healing. It is hard for families to accept that their loved one was in that much pain to take his own life and that by his own hands he chose the pain that his family is living with. It is even harder to accept that they will never have the opportunity to change the outcome. Some people view suicide as the ultimate act of selfishness; how else does one choose to die knowing that his family will be devastated by his absence? I personally am not comfortable standing on that side of the fence. I believe that a person who chooses suicide has to be in such a dark hole that he is not able to grasp how much pain his family will experience as a result of his actions. Depression has such a strong hold on them that they get tired of existing and ultimately just give up. In many suicide cases, the families are able to recall certain conversations and behaviors that signaled something was not right. Do not ignore the warning signs like depression, helplessness, hopelessness, impulsive and abusive behavior, talking or writing about death and suicide, withdrawing from family and friends and losing interest in favorite things. There are other signs to look for so do your research. Speak to a professional about ways you can help someone who might be struggling and exhibiting signs of defeat.

If you lost a loved one from suicide, please know that you cannot live the rest of your life held hostage by guilt, shame and defeat. People make unwise and unhealthy decisions not because they are unloved, but because they don't know who they are. They cannot see their strengths, only their weaknesses. Instead of celebrating their successes, they allow their failures to be magnified and entertain feelings of inadequacy and worthlessness. Every good parent raises their children to be respectful, kind and to make good decisions, but sometimes the kids miss the mark. Unfortunately, good parenting does not prevent children from making poor decisions. Your loved one's actions are not a bad reflection on you as a parent, spouse or friend. You cannot change what happened yesterday, but you can change your today by not allowing guilt to hold you back any longer. We only get one life to live, so choose to make the most out of yours right now. Just like your loved one chose his fate, you have to decide right now how you want the rest of your life to look. Believe it or not, you deserve to be happy and free from feelings of shame and defeat. Make today the day you turn it around. You can turn it around by being intentional about moving on and not allowing your experiences to trade places with your peace and your joy. Join a support group for people who have been affected by suicide or other loss. You may be surprised at how much comfort and strength you can find in these groups. You can also journal your feelings or go to lunch with a friend. You have to remind yourself that you are bigger than your pain. When negative feelings start to creep in, pick up a Bible and let your Creator remind you of how much He loves you. You are not at this place in your life by coincidence or by chance. Some of our greatest strength lies behind our pain and our struggles. If we throw in the towel too soon, the depth of that strength will never be realized. Just like a good pot of homemade soup, everything stays at the bottom of the pot until the heat is turned up. When the fire is the hottest, you will see those carrots, potatoes and corn start rising to the top. There are some things in us that will never come to the surface until the heat is turned up by way of our circumstances. Obstacles are like speed bumps, they were intended to slow us down, but never to stop us. We owe it to ourselves to keep running. Don't focus on the time clock, focus on the goal. Remember that the race is not given to the swift, nor is it given to the strong, but to the one who endures until the end. Are you an end runner or will you allow speed bumps to disqualify you from the race?

# HAVE YOU HEARD THIS ONE?

---

Let's face it. Death can make even a guy with tattooed lips and pierced eyeballs shake in his steel toed boots. They will strangle a rattle snake to death with their bare hands, but don't bring up death around them. You will hear more squealing than third graders on a roller coaster ride. They refuse to discuss it for more than a few minutes believing that the conversation brings with it bad luck. They believe that talking about it too long attracts death to them and nobody wants to remind death that they are still alive. I have heard it said many times that you are *never* supposed to say that a deceased person looked good dead. For example, "Boy, they really did a good job on Joe, he looked just like he was sleeping" or "That dress looked so good on Mattie, I hope they have me looking that good when I go!" As soon as those words are spoken (according to my sources) death puts out a hit against that person. One minute they are happily drinking a slurpee they bought from the corner store. Then they swallow and it goes down the wrong pipe and Bam! Just like that, they are gone. Just like poor old Joe and Mattie. I have also heard that when people dream about a deceased person that they will soon be joining them. Apparently, the dream is intended to warn you to get your affairs in order here on earth. It's your fault if you choose to ignore the signs. You have probably heard all of the ones about black cats and black birds, so I will spare you those details. There are two things that I have never claimed to be. One is a scholar and the other is a genius. But I feel confident enough to step out on a limb and say that those are all myths that have circulated throughout the ages. I have found that people make up strange stories and theories to make sense of the unexplainable. They accept whatever soothes them intellectually. People have done the same thing with God. Some believe that He is real while others cannot conceive such a being. Some people can accept Jesus, but not the heaven and hell concept. Some are comfortable with heaven, but not so much with hell. I am convinced that these beliefs (or lack thereof) gave birth to the many religions and faiths that exist today. So when people are uncomfortable with a particular thing, they tend to allow their imaginations to run free and unrestricted. Logic is placed on the back burner with the peas and carrots. Much of this stems from people not having a healthy understanding of death. They think that death is a random act that occurs by chance. They believe that at the start of everyday, the Grim Reaper summons his death angels and gives them the list of names of all who will die on that particular day. I hate to shatter your theory, but according to Psalms 139:16 all the days ordained for us were written in God's book before one of them came to be. God predestined the number of days that we would spend on this earth before we were born. No one is able to understand God's reasoning or rationale used to determine the times He set for any of us. Some babies die in the womb never having an opportunity to experience life. Others die having lived full lives. Instead of spending the remainder of my life trying to make sense of the process, I choose to spend it fulfilling the purpose that God placed in my life. What about you?

# WHERE WAS GOD?

---

Death can shake our foundational beliefs and even our faith. Some want to question why a God who is so loving and full of mercy allow something so devastating to happen in your life. It is hard to accept that instead of Him steering danger away, He permitted it to come to you. Ecclesiastes 3:1-8 (KJV) shares with us that "*To everything there is a season, and a time to every purpose under the heaven: A time to be born, and a time to die; a time to plant, and a time to pluck up that which is planted; A time to kill, and a time to heal; a time to break down, and a time to build up; A time to weep, and a time to laugh; a time to mourn, and a time to dance; A time to cast away stones, and a time to gather stones together; a time to embrace, and a time to refrain from embracing; A time to get, and a time to lose; a time to keep, and a time to cast away; A time to rend, and a time to sew; a time to keep silence, and a time to speak; A time to love, and a time to hate; a time of war, and a time of peace.*" God never promised that we would not experience hardships, sorrow and hurt in this life. He never assured us that our lives would be filled with happiness and pleasure exclusively. But He has made us some promises and we can be assured that He will fulfill every single one of them. God promises in Hebrews 13:5 (KJV), "*I will never leave thee, nor forsake thee.*" That tells me that no matter what we through in this life that He will be right there by our sides. Even when we can only feel the hurt and the pain, He is right there covering us with His peace and His love. In Psalms 23:4 (KJV) David shares with us, that "*Yea, though I walk through the valley of the shadow of death, I will fear no evil: for thou art with me; thy rod and thy staff they comfort me.*" David is facing a grim situation, but He is comforted by God's presence. God promises that we will be reunited with those in Christ who have departed from this life. Listen to Paul speaking to the church in 1 Thessalonians 4:13-14 (KJV), "*But I would not have you to be ignorant, brethren, concerning them which are asleep, that ye sorrow not, even as others which have no hope. For if we believe that Jesus died and rose again, even so them also which sleep in Jesus will God bring with Him."* There will be a great reunion and we will be reunited with all of our loved ones who went before us. We will never to be shaken by death or pain or heartache again. God promises in Matthew 28:20 (KJV) that *"I am with you always, even unto the end of the world. Amen."* I don't know about you, but even my closest friends have limitations and obligations that keep them from getting to me as quickly as I need them sometimes. But God is there in it all and through it all. David begged the question in Psalms 139:7-10 (NIV),

> *"Where can I go from your Spirit?*
> *Where can I flee from your presence?*
> *If I go up to the heavens, you are there;*
> *if I make my bed in the depths, you are there.*
> *If I rise on the wings of the dawn,*
> *if I settle on the far side of the sea,*
> *even there your hand will guide me,*
> *your right hand will hold me fast."*

Even in the midst of calamity we have a God who is there with us. God is not a god who is unfamiliar with our pain and our hurts. John 11: 33-35 tells us that when Jesus saw her (Mary) weeping, and the Jews who had come along with her also weeping, He was *deeply moved in spirit and troubled. "Where have you laid him? He asked. 'Come and see, Lord,' they replied. Jesus wept".* Notice that when Jesus saw Mary and the Jews grieving, He was moved. When we hurt, God responds to those hurts. He is moved to comfort us and give us peace even in the midst of our storms. This is a promise from God. In Philippians 4:7 (KJV) we find *"And the peace of God, which passeth all understanding, shall keep your hearts and minds through Christ Jesus."* I have seen people hit with massive blows of tragedy and witness God's peace carrying them through the fire. Peace is a gift from God that can be present in every stage of a believer's life. A person can be stricken with cancer, yet have a peace that is unexplainable, transcending our frail human minds. Peace says that even though my situation looks bad, I trust God for my life. Peace is a mindset that is unshakable and unwavering. The bigger the circumstance, the greater the peace. Our circumstances should never outweigh our peace. If it does, we can be assured that despair and desperation will plague our hearts and our minds. A perfect example of exhibiting peace in tumultuous times is found in the account of Job's life. Many of us are familiar with the story of Job and how he lost everything, his children, his property, and his livestock. Instead of his wife and friends supporting him through these losses, they all turned their backs on him. Listen to his response to his critical friends in Job 16:1-5 (NIV): *"I have heard many things like these; you are miserable comforters, all of you! Will your long-winded speeches never end? What ails you that you keep on arguing? I also could speak like you, if you were in my place; I could make fine speeches against you and shake my head at you. But my mouth would encourage you; comfort from my lips would bring you relief."* Job's friends ignorantly assumed that he had secret sin somewhere in his life that brought about all of his troubles. They refused to believe that all of these hardships would come to a sinless person. In the end, God condemned these friends who spoke against his servant Job. In Job 42:7-8 (KJV), *"And it was so, that after the LORD had spoken these words unto Job, the LORD said to Eliphaz the Temanite, My wrath is kindled against thee, and against thy two friends: for ye have not spoken of me the thing that is right, as my servant Job hath. Therefore take unto you now seven bullocks and seven rams, and go to my servant Job, and offer up for yourselves a burnt offering; and my servant Job shall pray for you: for him will I accept: lest I deal with you after your folly, in that ye have not spoken of me the thing which is right, like my servant Job"*. This is a reminder not to speak unwisely about another person's situation. You don't know what goes on behind the scenes and you could very well be bringing a curse against yourself. Job had indeed lived a righteous life before God and no wrong was found in him. He was a faithful man who had the opportunity to curse God and die. But instead Job's response in Job 1:21 was *"Naked I came from my mother's womb, and naked I will depart. The Lord gave and the Lord has taken away; may the name of the*

*Lord be praised.*" As a result of Job's reaction to his situation, he was restored. According to Job 42:12-17 (KJV), "*So the LORD blessed the latter end of Job more than his beginning: for he had fourteen thousand sheep, and six thousand camels, and a thousand yoke of oxen, and a thousand she asses. He had also seven sons and three daughters. And he called the name of the first, Jemima; and the name of the second, Kezia; and the name of the third, Kerenhappuch. And in all the land were no women found so fair (beautiful) as the daughters of Job: and their father gave them inheritance among their brethren. After this lived Job an hundred and forty years, and saw his sons, and his sons' sons, even four generations. So Job died, being old and full of days.*" I am certain that Job still grieved over the loss of his deceased children, but he allowed himself to move on and was able to create new memories that added to his life. So as you see, peace is a matter of choice. We can choose it over bitterness and resentment. Let me be clear here. Choosing peace does not mean that your suffering will be lessened in any way. It means that your situation won't define who you are as a person in Christ. Our experiences can shape us, but they shouldn't define us. For example, when a woman gives birth to or adopts a child, she becomes a mother. That is her experience. But that is not the totality of her as a person. If she defines herself as only a mother, what happens if that child dies or when he leaves home to pursue his dreams? Her identity is limited to a tangible thing, therefore when that thing is threatened, she is devastated beyond repair. I love my children dearly, but my identity is not dependent upon them or their actions. I am defined by my relationship in God. My identity is being a child of God who has given me a purpose to fulfill all of the plans that He has for my life. One of those plans is to tell the world that Jesus loves them so much that He died on a cross for their sins. Another is to be a wife to an amazing man. Another is to be a mother to three beautiful children. If a plan suddenly changes, I still have value and I still have worth because my identity is linked to the One who is unchangeable.

This is my prayer for you:

*"God, I come to you right now on behalf of my sister and my brother. They are at a crossroads in their life today and they are seeking divine direction. They have been devastated by life's experiences and are desperate to feel your Presence in their lives. I pray that you touch them right now, Almighty God. Open up their eyes, as you did Caleb and Joshua, so that they can see that You are with them and that you are bigger than their challenges. Renew their faith and their strength right now. Give them a limitless flow of grace and mercy to survive this season in their lives. Comfort those suffering from loss, restore love and peace back into their hearts and into their minds. I pray that you surround them with people who will encourage them and stand with them in their hour of need. I thank you God for not only hearing our prayers, but for responding to the needs of Your children. I thank you in advance for moving in the lives of Your people. I claim healing, restoration and peace. These petitions I ask in Jesus' name. Amen!"*

# FINDING YOU AGAIN

---

Right now you are at a crossroad in your life; a defining moment that will result in seven simple, but powerful letters. These letters define your experiences and signify your position here on this earth. They are the sum of your existence and write your life's story. These letters are either v-i-c-t-o-r-y or f-a-i-l-u-r-e. Many of you hate tests, not necessarily because they are hard, but because they represent what you have or don't have inside of you. Teachers know that in order to gauge what's on the inside of their students, they need to give them tests. They know not to go by what's on the outside, because the outside can be misleading. Many of you have faked your way for a long time, but when life throws you a pop quiz or a test, what's inside of you (or not) will determine whether you pass or fail. Many believers are living beneath their means as a child of the most high God. It is likened to having an envelope full of money, but refusing to use it. Your lights are disconnected, your refrigerator is empty and your car is about to be repossessed. You know that there is money in the envelope, but you are holding on to it until you really, really need it. This is how we are with our faith in God. We know that we have it, but we are looking for the right opportunity to unleash it. News flash. There is no time like the present. Unlike money in an envelope, we can never deplete our faith because our source comes from the Almighty; and the more we use it, the more He returns back to us. You are in the driver's seat today. You can go left or you can go right. No matter what direction you choose, those seven letters will be at the end of the road waiting for you. Some of you look into the rear view mirror and consider the option of putting the car in reverse. Moving backwards is familiar to you because you have done it your whole life. There are no new surprises. You know where every speed bump is and where every stop sign is posted. You have been down those roads many times before. You know what to expect as you drive down Pain Place, Regret Road and Anger Avenue. Some of you will choose to stay stuck in your grief because you are more comfortable with the pain, than you are with the unknown that lies ahead. Before you take your foot off of the brakes, let me share a few things that might help you. The very fact that you are holding this book assures me that you have survived. You have gone through the worst of it. It has happened, it's over and now it's time to move on. There are some of you whose lives have been shattered simply because you decided to follow your heart. Your intentions were good and you assumed that the person on the other end would reciprocate. But the more you gave, the less you became. By the time you realized the imbalance, you had spent a whole lot of time and a whole lot of life. You are bleeding, you are exhausted, but you are still here. There are many successful people who would not have realized their potential had they not tried "one more time". One more time unlocks opportunities and connections that are missed by those who choose to throw in the towel. Find out what *your* one more time holds for you. Moving ahead is possible. I know that resentment can be hard to shake especially if you lost a loved one as a result of another person's actions or if you were committed to a relationship that ended from mistrust. You can be angry, but do not let that define who you are. You must forgive and it only takes one person: you. Forgiveness is the best gift that you can give to yourself. This gift is for you, not the other person. Forgiveness is not easy, but it is possible. Remember Stephen's response to those who took his life. Forgiveness is liberating and it frees you from anger and bitterness. The other person is out there enjoying his life, while you are living like you are in prison. Make today the last day that you hold on to negative feelings. The rewards will be greater than the pain that is consuming your life. Start laughing again. It is purifying for your mind and body. Go out and catch a movie or read a good book. Call some of your wild and crazy *Christian* friends and go out and have a good time. (I had to emphasize "Christian" because I don't want any pastors upset with me.) Meet new people and start building new relationships. Sit down and compile a list of all of your favorite things. Mark them on a calendar and start enjoying your life again. Get an accountability partner that you can call when you find yourself looking in your rear view mirror. If they are a good friend, they will tell you how awesome you are and remind you that joy and peace are not optional for children of God, it is our right. Don't set unreal expectations for yourself. The pain from death will never disappear. The void of your loved one's absence will never be filled by anyone else, but going on is possible. As time passes, new memories can be created that will add meaning in your life. Don't cheat yourself by not reaching out to these opportunities. Also don't cheat other people by expecting them to live up to the standards of another person. That is not fair and it is not healthy. No one wants to be compared to another person or reminded how they are falling short in certain areas. This will turn people away from you. God designed our hearts with an unlimited capacity to love, but we have to take risks. There is a chance that you can be hurt and disappointed again, but there is also a chance that you will find happiness and fulfillment through relationships again. Remember as long as you look out of the rear view mirror, someone is deprived of knowing an awesome person and robbed of the opportunity to learn from you. You have a testimony that nobody can tell but you and people are dying because they need to hear that moving ahead is possible. There is somebody right now who is stuck and the only way they can be pulled out is by the hand of one who is familiar with pain and suffering. Everybody else has passed over them. They've been ignored and they've been cast aside. But they will trust you. Why? Because they know that you are the real deal. They can see your wounds; they see the scars that life has left on you. They know that you have been through hell and high waters, but you survived. They will trust you because they know that you would rather fall in the ditch with them than to walk away and leave them behind. How do I know so much? Remember my *friend*, Susie? That was me. (I'm surprised you didn't see this one coming). I was knocked down so hard that I stayed down. I built a wall around myself and refused to let anybody come near me. An unbelievable thing happens to a person when they stay down. Down starts to feel bearable to them. It starts to feel tolerable. They conform to their position and just exist. I existed for a long time. I had purpose, but I didn't know it. I couldn't understand it because I didn't know who I was. My identity was so wrapped up in what had happened to me that I could only associate with the hurt and the pain. I knew those two things better than anything else. When people stop fighting back guess what they do with all of that unused energy? They spend it rehearing their hurts and their failures. They think about what could have been. You always know when you're in the presence of somebody like that. They share their whole life story with you and the resounding message is "I'm the victim, I've always been the victim and I don't want to change anything in my life that will threaten my position as victim". Trust me, I have been there and done it quite a few times. I would still be right there had not some crazy people (family and friends) knocked down that wall and shared with me the same thing that I am sharing with you right now. There is life after pain. I am proof of that. I never thought in my wildest dreams that God would be able to use somebody like ~~Susie~~ me (I forgot that the cat was out of the bag). I was so battered and bruised, and filled to the brim with ugly and nasty experiences, but God uses me; and He will continue to use me as long as I am willing to go back in the trenches and pull out His forgotten ones. When my husband read my acknowledgements, he thought that I went a little overboard, but I told him that *all* of those people planted so many seeds in my life. Every success and every accomplishment is possible only because God used them to show me His love; and the best gift that we can give is to do for others what has been done for us. Plant a seed in someone else's life and watch how God makes good on the return in your life. The harvest out numbers the laborers, but we are charged to keep working. God uses those who are damaged and those whose stories may never be heard around the world. But their stories, like truth, are undeniable and change all who dare to listen.

# CULTURALLY SPECIFIC GRIEF DIFFERENCES

---

One of the worst mistakes that can be made is to assume that all grief looks the same. I have worked with many families from various ethnic and cultural backgrounds and have amazing insight. My aim is to provide you with *some* culturally specific grief patterns that I have witnessed over the years. This is not meant to be stereotypical or insensitive. Hopefully, it is an educational tool that provides a foundation that will enable you to show care and compassion to all who are in need regardless of race, culture or socioeconomic status. Please remember that this is not an exhaustive list and for a more in depth view, personal study is encouraged.

## AFRICAN-AMERICANS

African-Americans regard religion and family as the two largest factors that embody their rich and unique culture. At the first sign of a bad report, African-Americans usually cling to their faith with an unwavering stance. Many times I have seen these families completely discount a physician's report or prognosis, claiming that "the doctors only know so much, but God knows everything and we're waiting on His report." I have seen them ask for the ventilator not to be disconnected to allow God to perform a miracle. They also can be very mistrusting of hospitals and healthcare providers because of racism perceptions and experiments like the one done on the Tuskegee Airmen of Alabama. Usually all major decisions are made by the eldest person in the family. So for example, if elderly parents die and leave behind ten children, the eldest child will more than likely be at the forefront of decision making for the family, although advice may be solicited from other family members. Once they have accepted the fate of their loved one, a prayer is usually done around the bedside. Their displays of grief can often be described as animated, as they tend to be very expressive in their emotions. The funerals can last for hours and it is not uncommon for people to be "carried out" because they are unable to contain their emotions; interfering with the flow of the service.

## ASIANS

Asians have had a tremendous impact on American culture and they continue to evolve in unprecedented ways. Asians share many faiths, one of them being Buddhism. Buddhism has been described as a philosophical religion that is made up of unique beliefs and sacred traditions. Buddhist practicing Asians believe in reincarnation and believe that acts of goodwill will result in being elevated in body and/or in mind in the afterlife, as well as ensuring a smooth transition. Death is viewed as good or bad depending on the circumstances. For example, a good death is when one has lived a long life and has satisfied his life obligations. A bad death would be one that is untimely or violent. Asian males tend to make all of the decisions in the family. They can be trusting of healthcare providers and prefer to interact with males in superior roles. Asians tend to be reserved in their emotions and public displays of grief are minimal. There are specific mourning rituals that may be performed at the bedside of the deceased. Other rituals can last for up to three years after a person's death.

## CAUCASIANS

Caucasians consider family, their faith and reputation to be important elements in the fabric of their culture. When faced with life's challenges, the family typically makes decisions together as a complete family unit. Caucasians are extremely trusting of healthcare providers and are comfortable with asking questions regarding the care given to their loved one. Their reaction to a loved one's passing is usually seen by public displays of emotion. They may request that a pastor or chaplain come and perform a bedside prayer. Immediately following, they may request that their loved one's remains be prepared, so that the funeral home can start their embalming process to put their loved one to rest.

## HISPANICS

The Hispanic culture is very broad and diverse. They share a distinctive culture that is centered around their families, their faith and respect for their customs. It has been my experience that many Hispanic families embrace Catholicism and work hard at upholding the tenets of their faith. In times of adversity, the family unites and makes decisions that will benefit the family as a whole. In medical settings, Hispanic families can be very trusting of their healthcare providers. Upon learning of a loved one's death, they can be very demonstrative and expressive in their emotions. They also generally revert back to their native tongue when speaking amongst themselves. Oftentimes, Hispanic families will request that a priest come by to do the last rites for their loved ones. This gives them a lot of peace about the passing. Sometimes families will raise money in their communities to send their loved one's remains back to his country of origin.

## INDIAN/MIDDLE EASTERNERS

Indian and Middle Easterners have added an interesting and insightful perspective to life here in America. They place great emphasis on family, religion and culture. They can been described as modest and reserved. Indians/Middle Easterners can be suspicious in medical settings if they believe that the healthcare provider's intentions are questionable. All family decisions are made by the males in the family and the women are supportive in their roles. Indians/Middle Easterners prefer to interact with males in superior positions, as many of them feel that women are subservient to them. Indians/Middle Easterners tend to grieve quietly and are usually reserved in their emotions in front of those who are not family members. After a loved one's passing, families may request that the hospital bed or the remains be turned to face a specific direction. Death rituals may also be performed depending on how traditional the family is.

My friend, thank you for choosing to finish strong. Get excited about your future, because God is! He placed unique talents and abilities inside of you that nobody else has to fulfill a destiny that nobody else can. Stop comparing yourself to everybody around you. That same passion and capability lies within you. You were intricately and wonderfully made by the same hands that created the stars and the oceans. Our creator did not make any of us less than, for we were all made *good and very good*. He created us with our beginning and ending in mind; and put inside of us everything that was needed to finish strong. We have been given the choice of life and death. Please choose life. The world is depending on you to be you. In your darkest moments you can stand or you can kneel, as long as you find the strength to go on. Remember that love and compassion *always* triumphs over hatred, so give it liberally. I want to leave you right where we started, "*For I am persuaded, that neither death, nor life, nor angels, nor principalities, nor powers, nor things present, nor things to come, nor height, nor depth, nor any other creature, shall be able to separate us from the love of God, which is in Christ Jesus our Lord.*" (Romans 8:38-39, KJV)

I pray God's richest blessings upon you and your family!


*L. M. Ivy*